I0101091

Buff Body

12 Minute Full Body Workout

Buff Body
12 Minute Full Body Workout

Nikki Zeoli

Inspiration Publishers

The techniques and suggestions presented in this book are not intended to substitute for proper medical advice. Consult your physician before beginning any new exercise program. The Publisher assumes no responsibility for injuries suffered while practicing these techniques. The Publisher recommends those pregnant or nursing consult with their physician before beginning this exercise routine. For the elderly or those with chronic or recurring conditions such as high blood pressure, neck or back pain, arthritis, heart disease, and so on, please seek your physician's advice before using this book.

Copyright © 2016 by Nikki Zeoli

Original publication.

Cover and interior photos: by Charlotte Porzio

Back cover photo: by Johnathan Sloane

Printed in the United States of America

ISBN: 978-0-9977058-0-5

All rights reserved. No part of this publication may be reproduced or transmitted for commercial purposes without written permission of the publisher.

Inquiries regarding requests to reprint all or part of Buff Body should be addressed to Inspiration Publishers at the address below.

Other inquiries can be directed to:

Inspiration Publishers

20 Meeker Road

Westport, CT 06880

or

ZPublications@gmail.com

Dedication

To my greatest love – my husband Bert

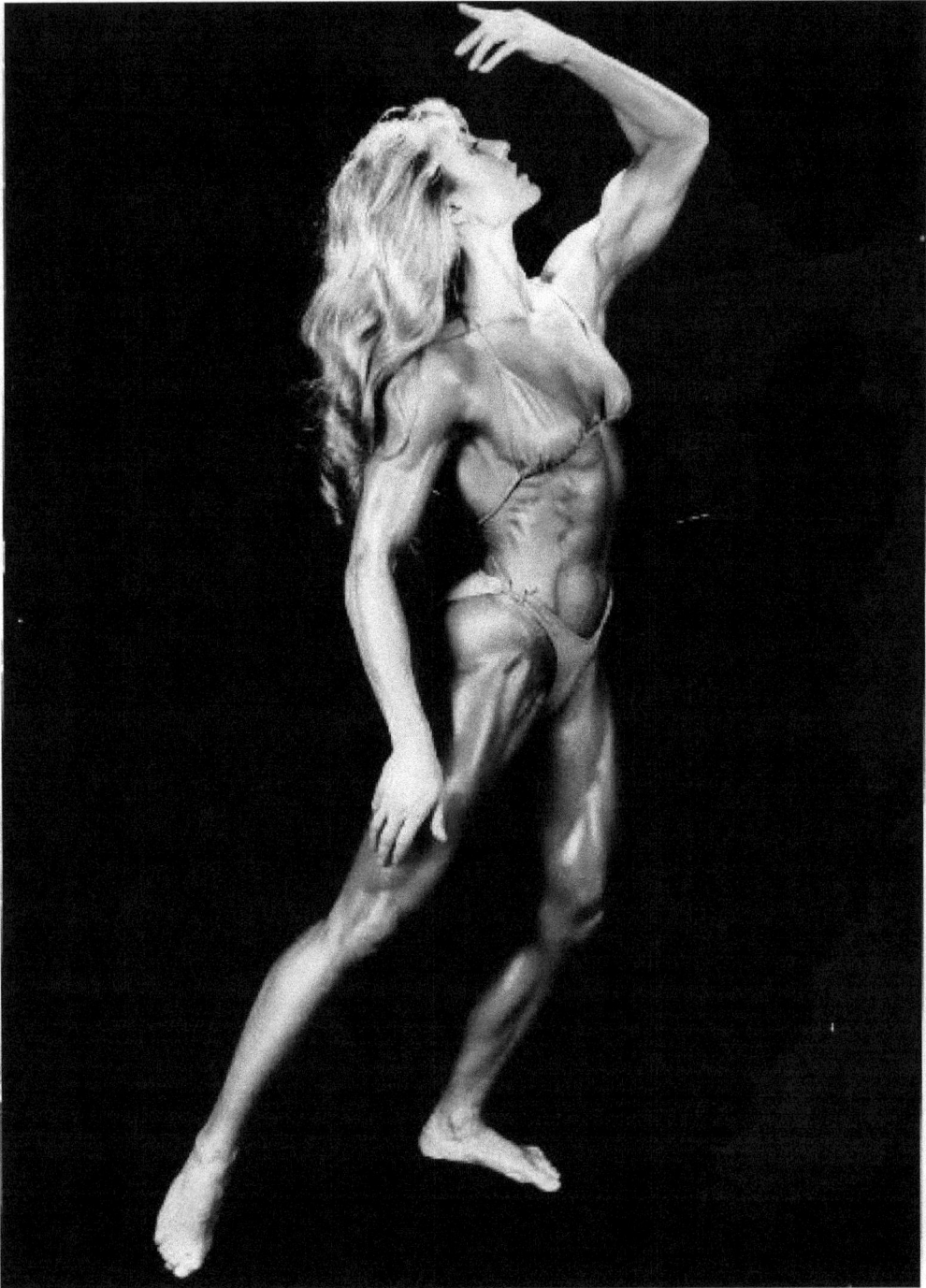

1993 National Champion

Table of Contents:

About the Author

Nikki Zeoli has been a professional fitness trainer for 25 years. She has instructed fitness pageant and bodybuilding contestants in workout design and implementation, as well as in make-up and presentation.

She is a past Overall Champion of the ANBC National Bodybuilding Competition, and took the fourth place prize as a professional bodybuilder in the 1993 World Natural Bodybuilding Federation National Championships. Nikki has competed in several national fitness competitions, including the 1997 Fitness America Miami Beach Championship. She has earned the Sportsmen of Westport (Connecticut) lifetime achievement award.

Her father, nationally renowned athletic director Nicholas Zeoli (Wilton High School, Wilton, CT), is a past president of the Connecticut Special Olympics. Nikki herself is a fierce advocate for children with special needs. She has worked with special needs youngsters in a variety of athletic endeavors in her home state.

She lives in South-Western Connecticut with her husband and three children.

FOREWORD

I love being fit – the way it makes me look and feel. Many ask "How do you have time to stay fit?" My answer is: Fitness is a "must" for me. It is an integral part of my personal identity. It's this perspective I maintain of myself - as a fit person - that compels me to make it true.

Raise your standard of yourself so that getting and staying fit is a "must" for you – not something you will "get around to" someday. Accept nothing less. Using the information in this book you will make it so.

After having children, I feared that I would lose my "fitness" identity. The workout in these pages is the result of the compelling "must" in my psyche to remain fit – to live up to my vision of who I am.

I don't have any more free time than anyone else. My first child was born severely disabled. I spent the first years of her life taking her to myriad doctor's appointments, physical therapy, speech therapy and occupational therapy. I was overwhelmed. My vision of myself as a fit person fell second to the "must" to do what was necessary to give my daughter the best chance at life.

For a few years I did get out of shape because I didn't think I had the time or the emotional strength to work out. This was unfortunate as it was precisely at that time that I most needed the physical and emotional benefits of exercise to handle life's challenges. I eventually forgave myself and got my body moving again while also working to care for my daughter, as well as my two other children born shortly thereafter.

The workout routine in this book is the result of my efforts to get fit during this busy and difficult time. Soon I had more energy and emotional stamina to do what was necessary to nurture all my children as well as create a fulfilling, passionate, and healthy life for myself (which benefits my entire family.)

"Just do it" the motto coined by Nike is stellar advice. Often we do not exercise because we feel overwhelmed, depressed or stressed. However, studies have clearly shown that even moderate exercise improves mood, increases stamina, creates emotional stability, and is a key factor in improving and maintaining a positive state-of-mind. So if we "just do it" – 12 minutes a day - we create a new, positive physical and emotional cycle of increasing proportions. A better life for ourselves and loved ones.

The routine outlined in this book will make a substantial difference in your body and health if followed diligently. It is a superior basic training method for our time-stressed lives. It lays a thorough foundation for the beginner, and increases already-developed levels of fitness. This workout stands on its own as the answer to getting and keeping your body fit and healthy.

For the adventurer, and person who wishes to push her or his fitness to a higher level, this system can be incorporated into a more exhaustive regime. For example, one or two days a week can be dedicated Buff-Body days. Another day or two can be at the fitness center using fitness machines. And yet another one or two days a week can be dedicated to yoga, martial arts, dance, swimming, or any other activity that moves the body and stimulates a training effect. Combining these variations can lead to extraordinary fitness levels.

When competing, I committed more time to working out and indeed did use several variations of training in order to get the most thorough workout possible to gain the competitive edge. While that level of training is not necessary for the non-competitor, it can be a fun challenge as fitness becomes a larger and more important part of your life.

Inspiration begins with the strong foundation in this book. From there, the possibilities, are endless.

A YOUNGER BODY

This is the Fountain of Youth! Exercise. Strength training exercise, in particular. It's like a magic pill that you can take any time to make you look and feel vibrant and healthy, live longer and with higher quality of life.

And the delicious secret is exercise doesn't have to be a long and painful process.

The advantages of strength training exercise are so abundant, I will not list them here as that would fill volumes. The following, however, is my list of favorite benefits that I have enjoyed over the years by regularly performing the exercise program described in these pages:

★ My weight has stayed the same even though my age keeps increasing.

★ My emotional state of mind is strong, passionate and positive.

★ My body is lean with tight muscle and not much fat.

★ I am told that my body still looks good.

★ I sleep like a baby every night!

★ My skin and eyes are glowing and healthy-looking.

★ I have great endurance to stay active and keep having fun.

★ My heart is healthy - with cholesterol levels better than a teenager's!

★ I enjoy a very high quality of life blessed with great health over the decades.

★ My balance remains excellent – which keeps me on my feet!

★ My bones are strong and joints flexible which keeps my posture firm and youthful.

★ Every day is joyful as I move with ease because my body is strong and agile.

Even a smoker, junk-food eater or person with other not-so-healthy habits or even addictions, will improve overall health, looks and metabolism just by performing strength training exercise regularly. That is how profound its effects are.

It makes your body younger.

THE CHALLENGES

Our lives are so busy that we do not have time to give ourselves this simple gift of exercise. This book delivers the information and opportunity to change that.

The sequence of exercises described herein is surprisingly convenient and effective in strengthening and shaping the major muscle groups of the body. The routine takes about 12 minutes to complete, and requires minimal equipment – making it easy to do almost anywhere. There are no excuses not to exercise!

As a mother of three school-aged children I swear by the effectiveness of this workout. My life is obscenely busy - I know yours is too - still I easily sneak the routine in during my day. When my daughter has physical therapy, I move to a corner of the room and do the workout. When my son is having his swim lesson, I go to a flat area of floor a few feet from the pool and do the routine. I sometimes sneak in a workout in my living room when my family is in bed (I definitely sleep better afterwards!). I have easily done it in hotel rooms when traveling, and even in my office.

At the age of 54, I frequently get compliments on the shape of my arms, calves, legs and overall figure. It always feels good to hear compliments because it confirms that my exercise routine achieves and maintains observable results.

Besides exterior benefits, this workout has truly kept me strong, agile, and feeling younger than my years. I have the energy to keep up with my kid's lives, spend quality time with my husband, maintain meaningful, fulfilling friendships, *and* write this book.

I marvel at how easy it is to maintain.

EVOLUTION OF THIS EXERCISE SEQUENCE

This workout routine evolved over several years. I was not consciously trying to put together a routine to publish. I was simply trying my best to keep my body young and healthy in the minimal free time I had.

By applying experience and knowledge I had gained from years of bodybuilding and professional fitness training, I developed, over time, the best way to fit into my day a comprehensive workout, requiring the shortest period of time, with a minimum of equipment. The result was this method of strength-training exercises (which includes relevant stretches). I still find it to be superior to any others.

By isolating all the major muscle groups of the body, this program systematically strengthens and balances the entire body – not just specific parts. This program works these major muscle groups:

1. Abdominals (Pilates bicycles)
2. Chest, or pectoral muscles (push-ups)
3. Thighs and buttocks (lunges)
4. Back or dorsal muscles (bent-over rows)
5. Upper front arm, or biceps (arm curls)
6. Shoulders, or deltoids (shoulder press)
7. Calf muscle or gastrocnemius (toe presses)
8. Back of upper arm, or triceps (triceps kick-backs)

For enhanced effectiveness and efficiency, the exercises are deliberately paired together, back to back. Working discrete muscle groups consecutively in this way allows you to perform the sequence without stopping, since each distinct muscle group has a rest while you work the opposing group. In the bodybuilding world we call these "super-sets."

Each set of "super-sets" is followed by stretches relevant to the muscles we have just worked.

As you are strength training with consistent intensity throughout the duration of the 12 minute workout, you also enjoy moderate to strong cardiovascular conditioning - another vital component of good health and fitness.

This program is easy-to-do and strengthens your whole body. A strong body burns more calories 24 hours a day, seven days a week.

Get ready to lose lumpy body fat and gain smooth firm muscles, strengthen your bones, move with youthful grace and posture, sleep better, look better and eat more if you want without affecting your shape.

ON YOUR MARK, GET SET. . .

Go barefooted or put on athletic shoes. Wear comfortable clothes. Place a mat (yoga mat is fine) or towel on the floor to do your work on. Have two pairs of dumbbells: one pair 5 pounds and one pair 3 pounds. When you are able to do the exercises with these weights easily for the required amount of repetitions, increase the weights one or two pounds at a time.

Perform this routine a *minimum* of twice a week. If you find it easy to fit in your schedule, doing it up to every other day will achieve quicker results.

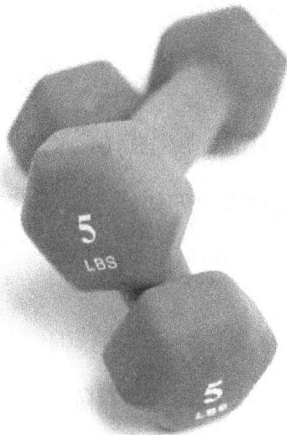

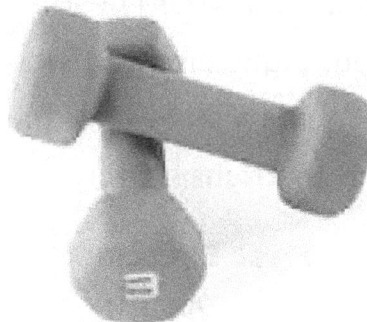

BEGIN ROUTINE

WARM-UP: We begin by loosening up the body from head to feet.

Head roll. Stand on mat. Relax shoulders, keep stomach tight, tuck pelvis under, knees slightly bent - not locked straight. Keeping shoulders stationary, roll your head slowly to the left – left ear toward left shoulder, then let your head drop forward - chin toward your chest. Next, roll head to the right so that your right ear reaches towards your right shoulder, then look up toward ceiling (see **figure A**). Repeat. Reverse the direction, doing two head rolls in the opposite direction.

Shoulder roll. Bring your shoulders forward and up (toward your ears), and then let them roll back and down. Repeat circle twice more. Reverse direction and do three shoulder rolls (see **figure C**).

Torso twists. Twist your chest left, letting arms swing naturally in the same direction. Your right arm will wrap around the left side of your waist (see **figure B**). Then twist toward the right, swinging your left arm so that it wraps around the right side. Repeat five more times.

Transition to First Exercise: Bend your knees in a squatting position, put your hands on the floor in front of your feet (see **figure D**). Slowly straighten your legs to a point that you comfortably can (see **figure E**) feeling a stretch in the backs of your legs. Relax your head and arms and let them hang down in front of your legs. Bend down again in the squatting position and repeat three times. Slowly unroll your spine - think of doing this one vertebra at a time - until you are back to a standing position.

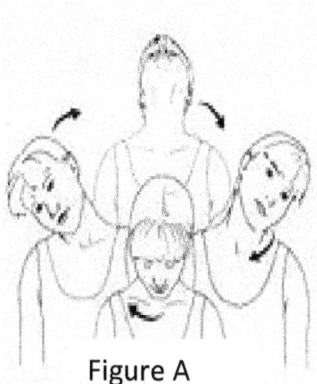
Figure A

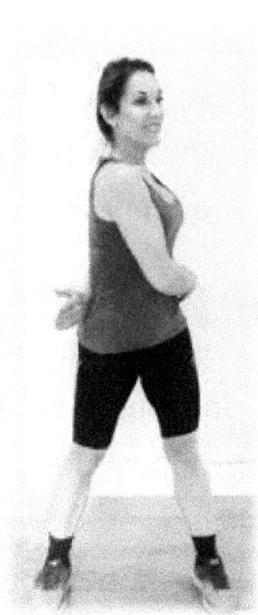
Figure B

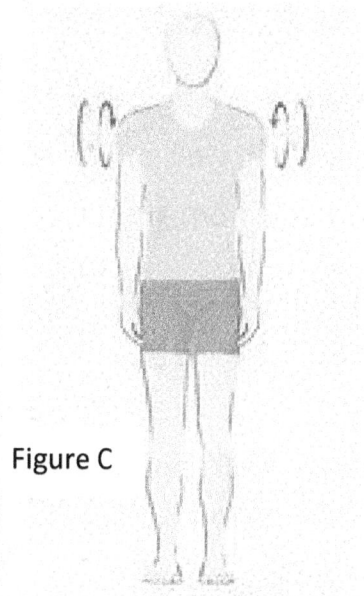
Figure C

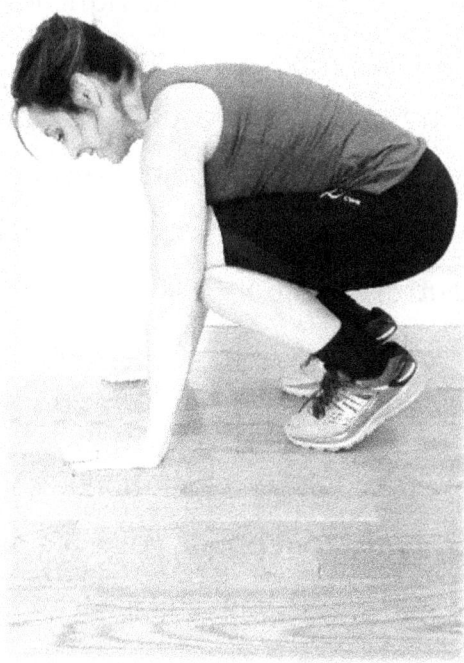
Figure D

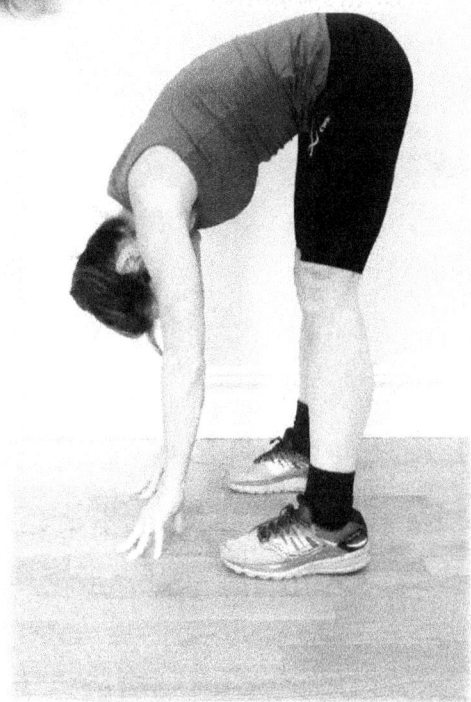
Figure E

EXERCISE I

Pilates Bicycles: Strengthens your entire abdominal wall – working the front wall of the stomach and oblique muscles (abdominal muscles running from your sides at an angle to your front abdominal wall).

Lie on your back, with your head resting on the pads of your fingers (see **figure 1A**). Do not lace your fingers behind your head as this may force your head forward and put a strain on your neck. Keeping your lower back flat against the floor, bring your left knee in toward your chest, at the same time lift your head and right shoulder, twisting from your waist and reaching the right elbow toward your left knee (see **figure 1B**). Hold for a slow count of two. As you do this, the right leg stays straight and hovers just about five inches above the floor. Switch sides – reaching your left elbow to your right knee. This counts as one repetition. Continue with the exercise, alternating sides, being sure to keep lower back against floor to protect it, and head resting on the pads of fingers, keeping your neck in a neutral position. Aim for 30 repetitions. If you absolutely cannot do 30, go for at least 20. If, in the beginning, you must stop and rest, do so, briefly, and continue to 20.

Cobra Stretch: When finished with the Pilates Bicycle repetitions, roll over on to your stomach. Push up on your hands, keeping your pelvis on the floor, looking forward, and stretch your abdominal muscles (see **figure 1C**). Go directly to the next exercise.

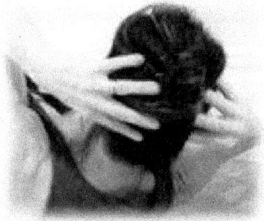

Figure 1A

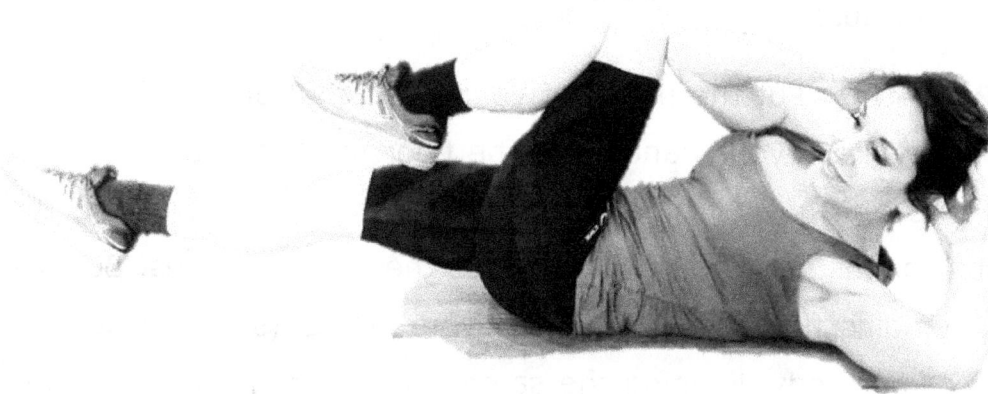

Figure 1B

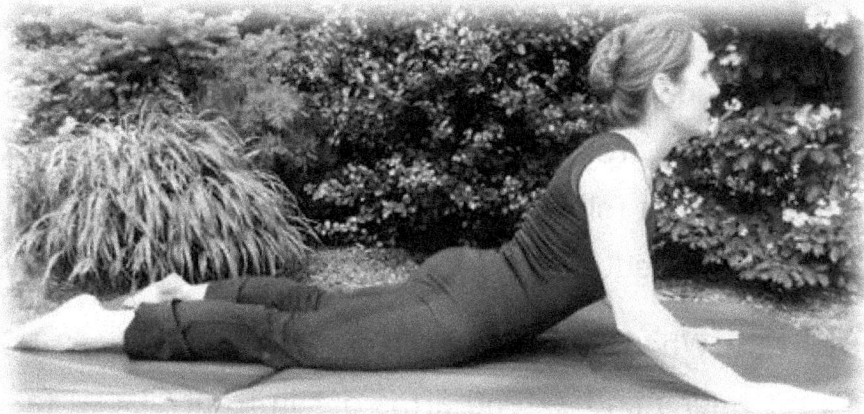

Figure 1C

EXERCISE II

Push-Ups: Works the large muscles of your chest, the front of the shoulders, and abdominal muscles.

First, determine which type of push-ups you are capable of doing. Most men, depending on age and health, can do military push-ups. Many women can too – and if you can, than do. If they are too difficult, do the modified pushups.

Military Push-Ups: Put the palms of your hands flat on the floor near your shoulders. Press your hands into the floor so that your torso and head move up and away from the floor. Concentrate on pressing the heels of your hands into the floor to isolate the chest muscles. Be sure your back remains flat and in line with your pelvis (see **figure 2A**). Slowly lower your body, keeping the same alignment of your back and pelvis, until your nose almost touches the floor (see **figure 2B**). Do not let any other part of your body that isn't already touching, touch the floor. As you push up and lower down (one repetition), be sure your elbows bend out away from your body at a 90 degree angle. Continue slowly and deliberately (slow count to two up, and slow count to two down) for 12 to 16 repetitions.

Praying Stretch: When finished, sit back onto your calves, lower your torso onto your thighs and extend arms out in front of you (see **figure 2E on page 29**) feeling a stretch in your arms and chest.

Roll onto your back and immediately repeat the **Pilates Bicycles**. Right away, roll onto stomach again and repeat one more set of **Push-Ups**.

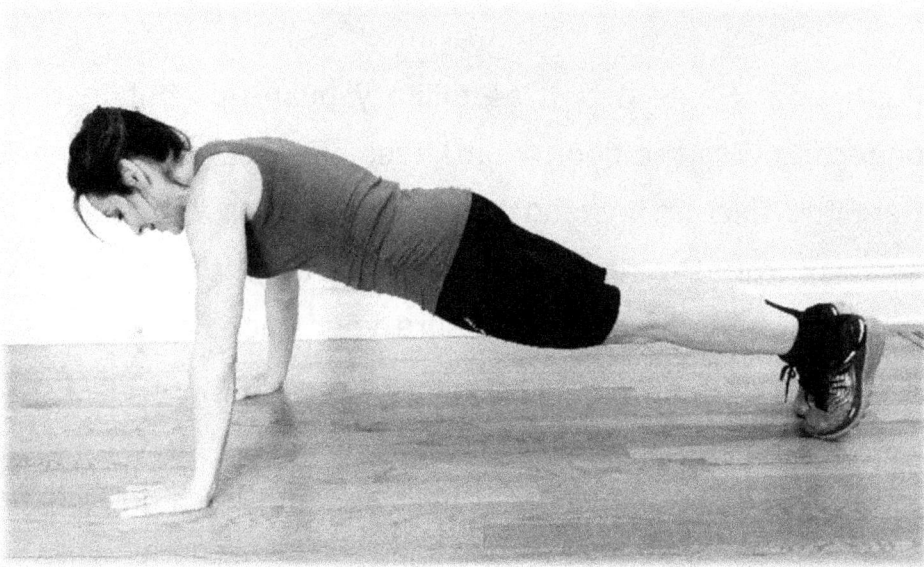

Figure 2A

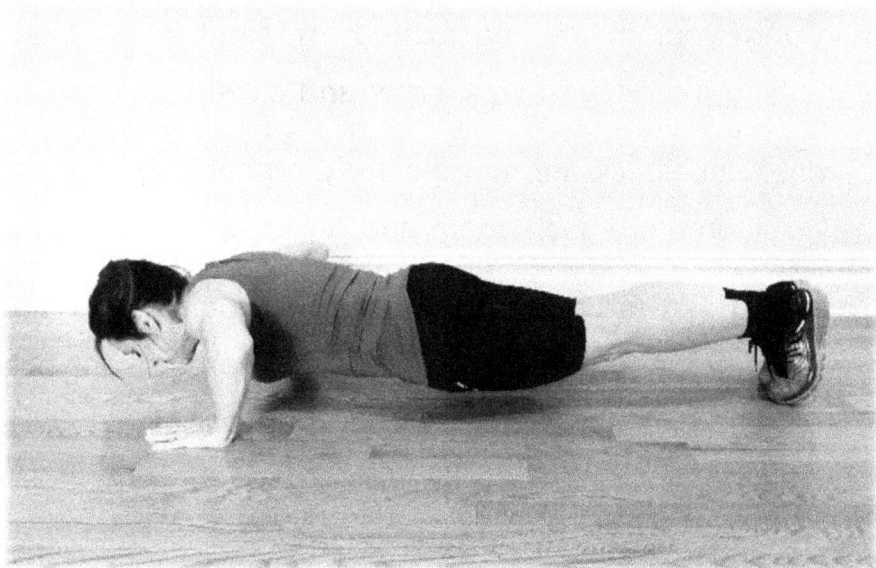

Figure 2B

Modified Push-ups: Same action as military push-ups but instead of your feet connecting with the floor, your knees connect (see **figure 2C**). Your knees are the fulcrum instead of your feet. Press your torso and head up and away from the floor by pressing through the heels of your hands to isolate the chest muscles. Be sure your back remains flat and remains in line with your pelvis. Slowly lower your body down, keeping the back/pelvis alignment, until your nose almost touches the floor. Do not let any other part of your body that isn't already touching, touch the floor. As you push up and lower down (one repetition), be sure your elbows bend out away from your shoulders (see **figure 2D**). Continue slowly and deliberately (count to two up and two down) for 12 to 16 repetitions.

Praying Stretch: When finished, sit back onto your calves, lower your torso onto your thighs and extend arms out in front of you (see **figure 2E**) feeling a stretch in your arms and chest.

Roll onto your back and immediately repeat the **Pilates Bicycles**. Right away, roll onto stomach again and repeat one more set of **Push-Ups**.

Transition to next exercise: Bend your knees and bounce, then straighten your legs letting your head relax in front of your legs. Again bend knees and bounce, bounce and stretch again (see **figures D and E on page 23**). Roll body up, think of stacking one vertebra on top of the other to a full standing position.

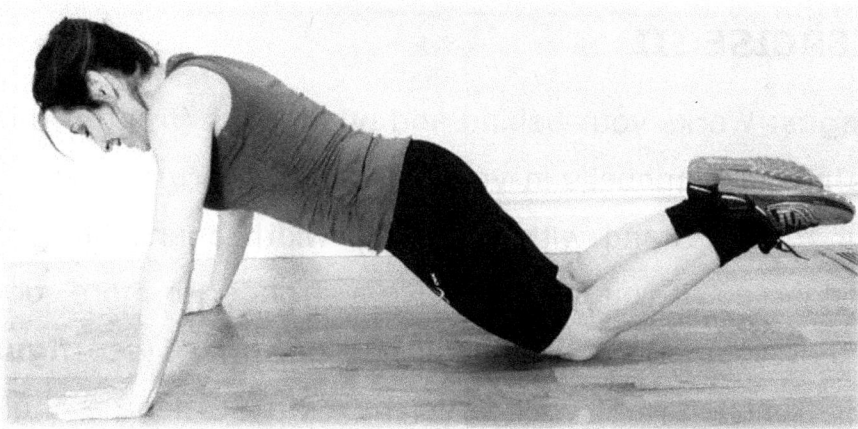

Figure 2C

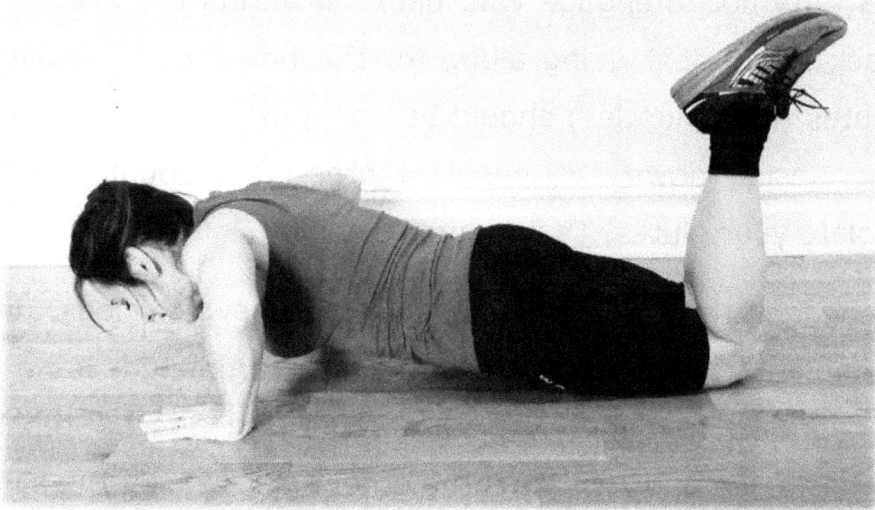

Figure 2D

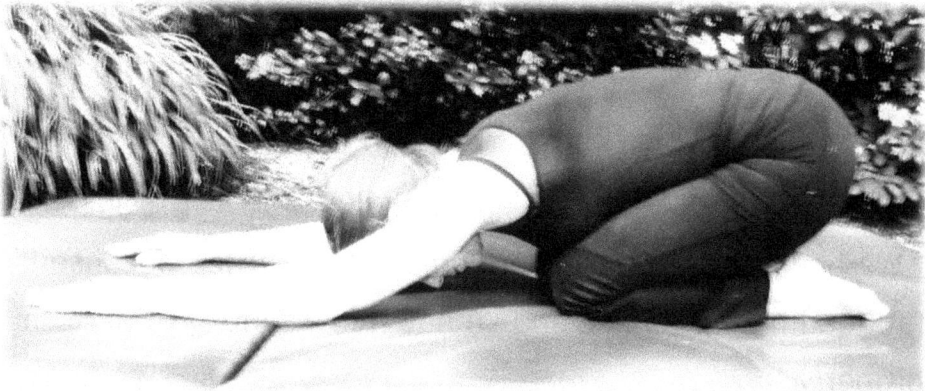

Figure 2E

EXERCISE III

Lunges: Works your behind and quadriceps (front of thighs). Hold the five-pound dumbbells in your hands, your arms should be hanging by your thighs. Stand with knees hip width apart. Step back with your stronger leg (if you feel you have a stronger or more coordinated leg)* so that your legs make an upside down "V" (see **figure 3A**). Bend your front leg until your knee makes a 90 degree angle (see **figure 3B**). Try not to engage your back leg during the exercise. Think of the back leg as just going along for the ride. Your front leg's thighs and glutes (butt muscles) should be doing most of the work. Press back to the upside down "V" position, pressing through your heal to help isolate your glutes. That is one repetition.

Repeat with the **same** leg. Do not switch legs until you have completed 16 to 20 repetitions. Once completed, bring your back leg forward so that feet are again hip width apart. Step back with the opposite leg and repeat on the other side, exactly the same way.

With lunges, you are simultaneously strengthening your quadriceps muscles as well as the glutes. The lunge is the best all-over leg exercise for strengthening and shaping the behind and legs – for both men and women.

*We begin the exercise working the weaker leg because it is less fatigued from exercise and so has more control to perform the exercise properly.

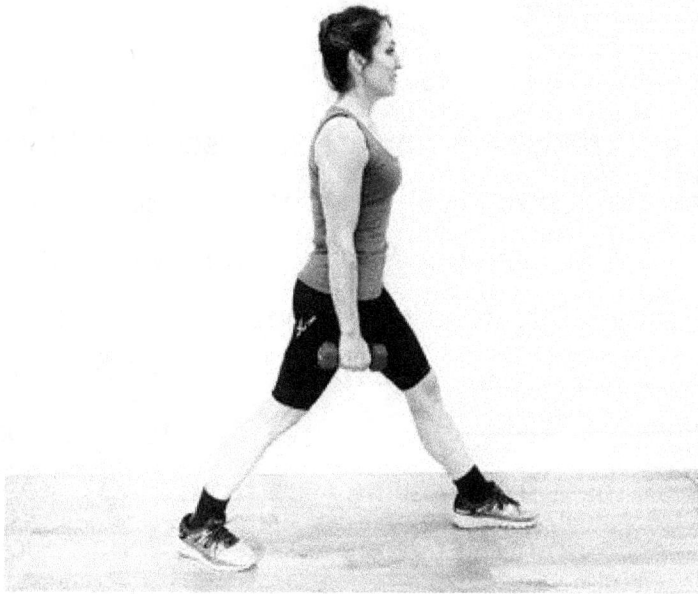

Figure 3A

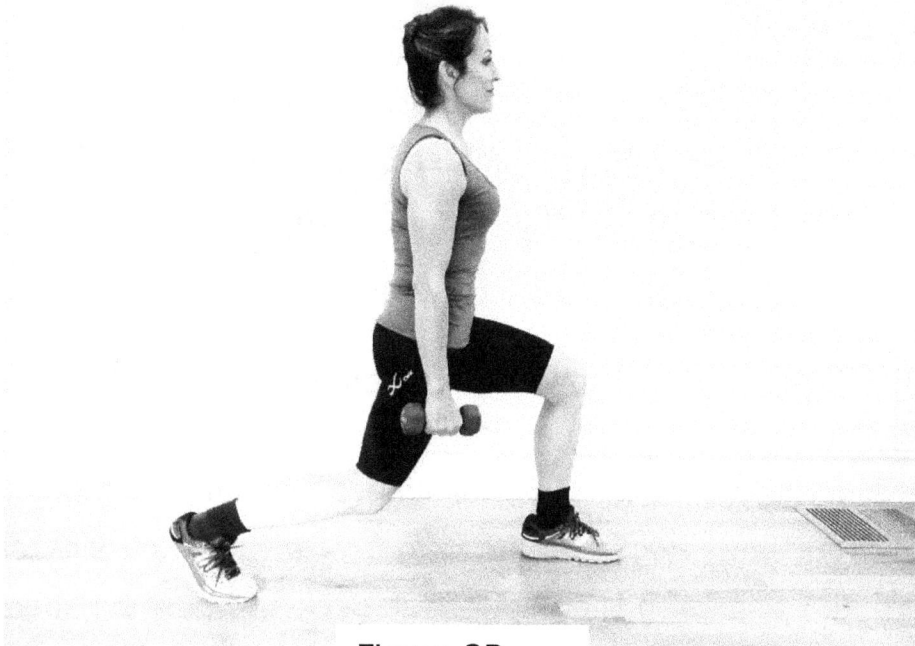

Figure 3B

EXERCISE IV

Bent-Over Row: Strengthens your back muscles. Hold your three-pound or five-pound dumbbells in each hand – keep your thumb on the same side of the bar as your fingers. Start with feet hip width apart, knees slightly bent, bend body from the waist so your torso is just about parallel to the floor (see **figure 4A**). Holding dumbbells with your wrists facing each other, lift the weights by lifting your elbows straight up toward the ceiling (see **figure 4B**). Keep your arms by your sides – do not let elbows "chicken wing." Slowly lower the weights straight down. This is one repetition. Be sure to keep your stomach muscles tight for support of your lower back. Repeat this exercise slowly and deliberately (slow count to two up and two down) for 12 to 16 repetitions.

Once completed, go back to the preparatory stance for **Lunges**. Use the heavier of your two sets of weights. Step back with your weaker leg and repeat another full set of lunges on each side.

Immediately repeat the **Bent-Over Rows**.

Transition: **Quadriceps Stretch**: With one hand, hold on to something stable, like a table, a door handle, or sturdy shelf. Bend whichever leg you used to begin your lunges so that your heel goes up towards your butt. Hold on to that foot with the same side hand (see **figure 4C)** think of pulling your knee back and pushing your hip slightly forward - you will feel a stretch in the front of your bent leg. Hold for a slow count of 20 then stretch the other leg the same way.

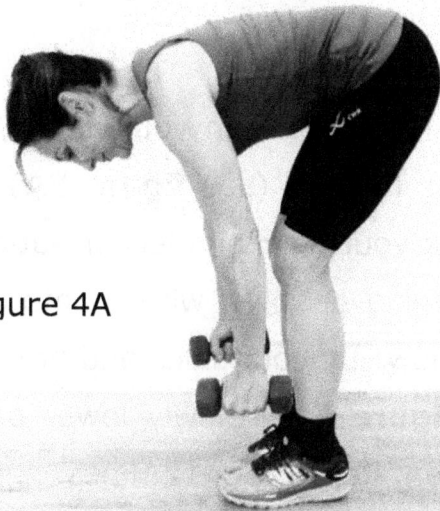

Figure 4A

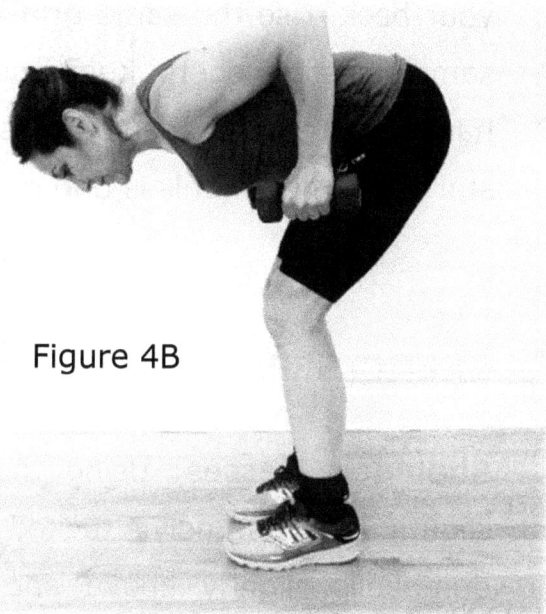

Figure 4B

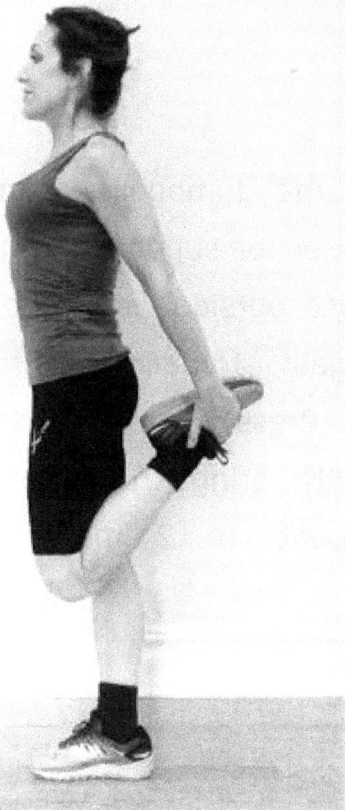

Figure 4C

EXERCISE V

Biceps curls. Stand with the lighter dumbbells in your hands, arms down at your sides and palms facing forward (see **figure 5A**). Keep your stomach muscles tight and tuck your pelvis under for support of your back. Use the same grip as bent-over rows, with thumb on the same sides as fingers. Keep your elbows by your sides and bring your hands up to your shoulders (see **figure 5B**). Slowly lower back to starting position. This is one repetition. Repeat 8 – 12 times.

EXERCISE VI

Shoulder Presses: Using the same dumbbells, stand with knees slightly bent and pelvis tucked under for support of your back. Bring dumbbells slightly above and just outside your shoulders, palms facing forward (see **figure 6A**). Again, stomach stays tight and pelvis tucked under for support of back. Press your hands straight up and together (see **figure 6B**). Slowly bring them back to starting position. This is one repetition. Repeat 8 to 12 times.

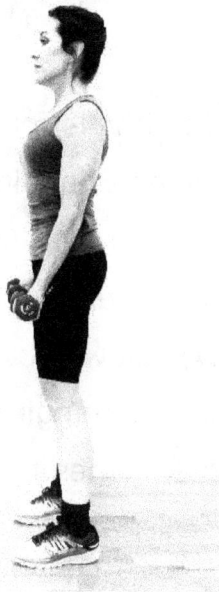

Figure 5A

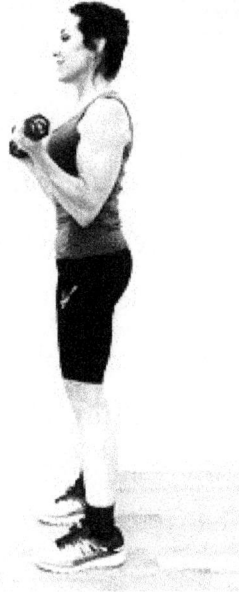

Figure 5B

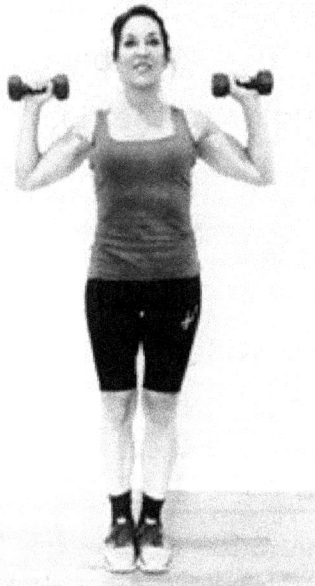

Figure 6A

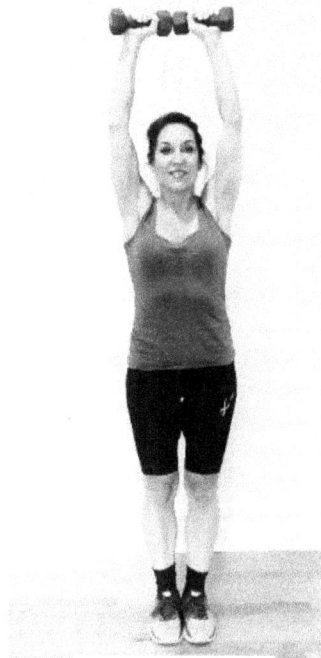

Figure 6B

EXERCISE VII

Toe Presses: Strengthens calf muscles. No dumbbells for this exercise, at least to start. Find a step of some sort. A stair or a landing will work. Put the balls of your feet on the edge of the step. Your mid-foot and heel will be hanging off the edge (see **figure 7A**). Slowly press up onto the balls of your feet like going on "tip toe" (see **figure 7B**). Slowly lower back through the original position and past so that your heels are hanging below the balls of your feet. This is one repetition. Repeat 8 to 12 times.

EXERCISE VIII

Triceps Kick-backs: Strengthens back of upper-arms. Hold the smaller dumbbells in your hands. Start from standing position, feet about hip width apart. Bend knees slightly, so they are softly bent, then bend from the waist so your torso is just about parallel to the floor. Your body is now in the same position as beginning the bent-over rows (see **figure 8A**). Keeping your elbows locked in place, extend your lower arm straight back – feeling the muscles in the backs of your upper-arms working (see **figure 8B**). Again, keeping your elbows in place, slowly lower your arms back to the beginning position. This is one repetition. Complete 12 to 16 repetitions.

Repeat the last four exercises (V – VIII) again in the same order. Now you are done.

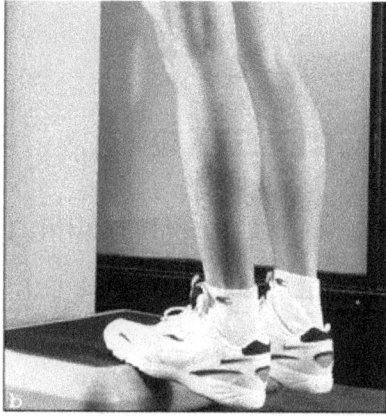

Figure 7A

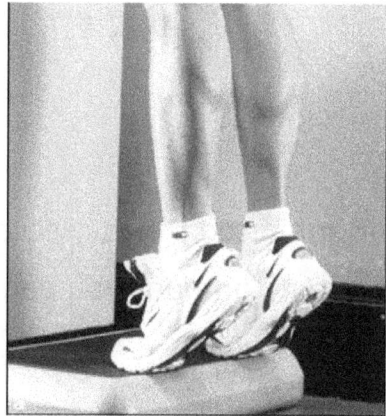

Figure 7B

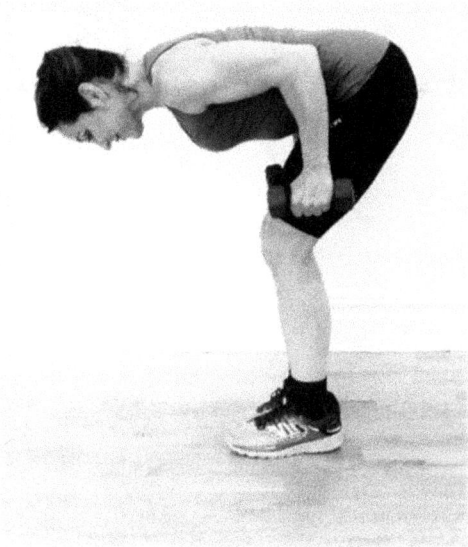

Figure 8A

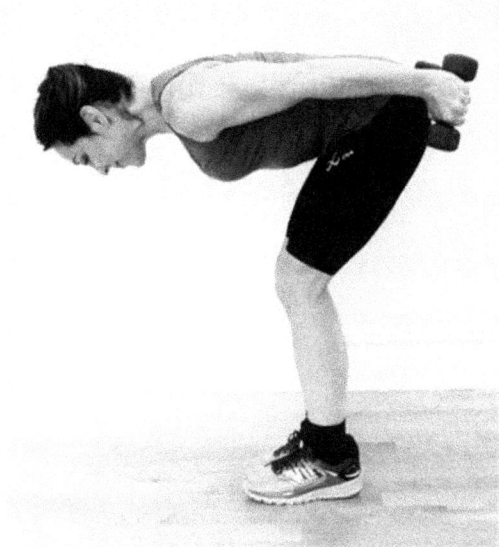

Figure 8B

PROGRESSING

For enhanced fitness, accompany this strength training routine with daily walking. Any amount you can fit in. Start with at least ten minutes. Walk fast and with purpose.

After you get used to doing these exercises and feel comfortable and confident with them, increase the weight. Usually the bent-over rows increase with two or three-pound increments. Lunges with three to five-pound increments. Curls one pound. Triceps and shoulders one to two-pound increments.

12 minutes = full body workout = happy and healthy body.

www.ingramcontent.com/pod-product-compliance
Lightning Source LLC
Chambersburg PA
CBHW051348290326
41933CB00042B/3331